No More Sickle Cell Crisis

A Bone Marrow Transplant Success Story
Based on a true story

Chy Butler, Pharm.D., RPh.

Copyright © 2018 Chy Butler

All rights reserved.

ISBN:9781729365076

Acknowledgement

Thank you! Dr. Bhatia, the entire transplant team, nurses and child life department at Morgan Stanley Children's Hospital, without their dedication and hard work, there would be no success story.

To my family, I am always humbled by your unending support. I love you all.

To my children; Isabelle and Gabriel; your love for each other inspires me.

To my husband, thank you for supporting all my dreams.

To my church family, thank you for all the prayers, texts and phone calls.

To anyone affected by sickle cell disease, you motivated me to share my story of healing and hope. You motivate me to strive to generate awareness.

Thank you germancreative for my cover page design.

Introduction

Jane sat on the bed next to Gabe. She watched as he received a transfusion of fresh bone marrow in plasma through one of the branches in his central line. This fresh bone marrow was donated a week ago by his big sister Angel. If this procedure works as intended, Gabe will no longer have sickle cell disease.

Chapter One

August 30th, 2012

Sharp pains woke Jane from her sleep. "I must be in labor;" she thought, "why can't you wait one more day Gabe?"

Slowly, she rolled her body to the edge of the bed, placed one foot on the carpeted floor and then the other. Taking a deep breath, she lifted her rotund belly off the bed. Just like her first pregnancy, this one came with a ton of extra weight.

"I need to hurry up and do some house chores;" she thought. "Gabe, you need to come out quick and painlessly;" she spoke to her belly. This was her daily ritual; conversations with Gabe; still in her belly, making his presence known with his frequent kicks.

Grabbing her phone from the night stand, she set a timer to track her contractions. After ten minutes with no notable contraction, she set about her usual morning routine.

Jane took a long hot and steamy shower, brushed her teeth and slowly made her way downstairs in search of food.

"This boy is definitely different from his sister;" she mumbled to herself, "I am starving!"

In the refrigerator was last night's leftovers; a few lamb chops, asparagus and curry quinoa. Throwing everything into a glass Tupperware, she set the oven on three hundred and fifty degrees for ten minutes. Smiling, she surveyed the dining area and living room. Everything was exactly as she left it last night.

Angel; her two-year-old daughter, had a sleepover at Grandma's house last night.

Jane's breath hitched as she was overcome by yet another contraction. She had her cesarean section scheduled for the very next day. Holding onto the kitchen counter, she tried to catch her breath by slowly inhaling and exhaling. She soon found herself reflecting on how hard she worked with Jide, to prepare Angel for the arrival of her little brother. Angel's favorite preparation video was that of Dora the explorer. In this video, Dora's mom was expecting twin boys. Angel watched this video at least once a day for the past four months. She also saw images of Gabe during Jane's antenatal visits. Angel could not wait to meet her brother.

"Mummy, do you think you'll have twins next time?" She randomly asked.

Jane just smiled. No need to engage her two-year-old chatterbox in a lengthy conversation on why this baby, was most likely going to be her only sibling.

Just then, the oven timer went off. Jane waddled to the oven, grabbed her morning feast and sat down to devour it. After having two trimesters of terrible morning sickness, she truly relished the huge appetite that came with this third and thankfully, final trimester. The weight gain on the other hand, that, she will handle after the delivery.

Four hours later, the contractions came back with a vengeance. She could hardly catch her breath in between each wave. She called her Obstetrician, when she felt certain that it was indeed, the beginning of labor.

"I feel like I'm in labor," she told the receptionist; Anna.

"Hold on for Doctor D", the receptionist replied.

Doctor D came on the phone.

"How far apart are these contractions you are feeling?" He asked.

"They are less than five minutes apart and these contractions are getting really painful;" Jane panted.

"Sounds like your son is ready to come out." Doctor D responded.

"Ok, head to the hospital. I will meet you there." He instructed.

Jane called Jide immediately.

"Where are you?" She asked as soon as he picked up his cellphone.

"I am on my way home;" he replied. "What did the doctor say?" He asked.

"He said it's time to head to the hospital." Jane responded.

"Great! Hang in there, I'll be there in less than ten minutes." Jide said before he hung up.

Jane slowly strolled around the living room. Her hospital bag was packed weeks ago. She was ready to leave for the hospital. Unconsciously, she strolled into the kitchen and grabbed a bag of nacho chips.

She was just about to bite down on the last chip, when Jide came home.

Sprinting up the stairs, he stopped abruptly when he saw Jane.

"Why are you eating that?" He asked, grabbing the hospital bag from the dining room table.

"I was hungry!" Jane snapped as she ate the final chip.

"Well, that snack is going to bring you a whole lot of pain now." Jide shook his head, wearing a troubled expression.

"The anesthesia team will wait for at least eight hours, for that bag of chips to digest. Especially if you end up with another cesarean section."

Jane swallowed dejectedly.

"I might as well eat a full meal." She teased.

That earned her a glare from her husband.

Chapter Two

Nine Hours Later

The soft angelic cry of a baby hit the longing ears of his parents.

"This cesarean section feels longer than the first one I had, two years ago with Angel." Jane thought.

After waiting for approximately eight hours for the bag of chips to digest, battling different waves of painful contractions and gulping down the nastiest tasting medication ever; to prevent vomiting, Jane was finally in the operating room.

Tears filled her eyes as Jide brought their baby over.

"He is so beautiful." she cooed.

"My dream has come true." She murmured to no one in particular. Exhausted from almost nine months of carrying this little watermelon in her belly, she fell asleep.

Chapter Three

Wake Up!

Jane's eyelids felt as heavy as iron rods. She tried to open them but failed. She willed them to open and they refused. "Darn these anesthetics," she complained.

"They definitely make labor pain a bit bearable but waking up, is very stressful."

She dozed off again.

Waking up the second time around, she slowly opened her eyes. Looking around, she saw a few blurry images. Struggling to focus on a single object, she squinting her eyes and spotted a nurse. Random thoughts started flying through her mind.

"How is the baby?" She tried to ask.

No sound came out of her mouth. After several failed attempts to speak, she forced herself back to sleep.

"I will try this again in another hour;" she thought.

She woke up again. This time Jide was watching her closely.

"I must have slept for longer than an hour," she thought.

Her words where slurred and slow as she fired questions at her husband.

"How is the baby? Does he have ten fingers and ten toes? Does he have baby teeth like the doctor thought he would?"

One question at a time Baby! Jide laughed.

"Gabe is fine. No! He does not have any teeth", Jide laughed, humor lighting his eyes.

Jane sighed, relieved.

Jide looked at her, with pride in his eyes.

"Gabe is just perfect." He smiled.

"But,' he paused, "Doctor D says he's a bit jaundiced. He's getting light therapy now."

Jane's heart skipped a beat. Jaundice! She searched her brain, trying to remember if Angel was born jaundiced as well. There is something about going through labor multiple times, you just can't help comparing experiences. However, Jane's brain was too muddled.

"God, please don't let him have sickle cell disease," she suddenly prayed.

"Does God answer this kind of prayer?" She pondered.

A few hours later, the nurse brought Gabe to be breastfed. Like his sister, he was going to be exclusively breastfed. Jane examined her son closely.

"He is so handsome." She thought yet again.

His hair was light brown and curly.

"He does not look too yellow to me," she mused, pushing down the wave of panic that was beginning to take momentum in her belly.

"I will just think positive," she counseled herself. Picturing Gabe in her head as a young strapping architect.

Chapter Four

Sibling Love

Jide brought Angel to visit Gabe at the nursery.

He excitedly pointed out a baby in the nursery. "That baby in the middle crib is your brother!" He said proudly.

The excitement was contagious. Waving at her baby brother through the glass window, Angel turned to Jide.

"When can we take him home, Daddy?" She asked.

"In a few days, my Princess. Let's go see Mummy." Jide replied.

Grabbing her Daddy's hand, they walked towards Jane's room.

Jane's hospital room was big and spacious. Angel especially loved the hospital bed. She loved pressing the button that slowly changed it from a bed to a chair. She sat on Jane's bed, looking at the contents of her food tray with interest. Finally, she settled on a cup of apple juice.

"I like this room, Mummy." She pronounced.

"When will they bring Gabe here? I want to play with him." Angel asked.

As if on cue, a nurse arrived with Gabe in his little crib.

"He's crying." She smiled. "He must be hungry."

Jane fed Gabe, then patted his back until he burped. He soon fell fast asleep.

"Can I hold him a little?" Angel asked.

"Sure, my little love," Jane said. "Just place your arm like this." Jane positioned Gabe in Angel's arms.

"He is very quiet." Angel observed. "Mummy, why is he sleeping so early? It's not bedtime yet. It's daytime!" Angel observed.

"Babies sleep a lot;" said Jane. "They have a lot of growing to do."

"Did I sleep a lot when I was a baby?" Angel asked.

"You definitely did!" Someone responded from the doorway.

"Grandma! Grandpa!!" Angel screamed, her little vibrant voice echoing in the halls.

"Come and see little Gabe. He just ate and now he is sleeping."

Grandma and Grandpa washed their hands. Grandma carried Gabe. She cooed and rocked him, gushing like most loving Grandmothers do. Grandpa beamed with pride, and placed the large bouquet of flowers by the bay window.

"Grandpa, did you forget the blue teddy bear I picked for Gabe?" Angel called out.

"How could I?" He replied. He pulled out the big fluffy blue teddy bear from a large paper bag. It was sealed in clear plastic wrapping.

Angel ran and took it from him. "I'll place it right …here."

She searched around for the perfect spot and placed it at the feet of Jane's bed. Satisfied with her work, she started humming a song from "The Sound of Music".

Soon, her sweet voice could be heard down the hall.

"Let's start from the very beginning…" She sang.

"You belong on Broadway;" a nurse passing by, stopped to tell her.

"I know." She replied, smiling.

Chapter Five

Discharged

Gabe and Jane were discharged three days later. Gabe was circumcised and ready to go home. They had to follow up with Gabe's pediatrician in a few days, to keep an eye on his jaundice. This was a precaution to make sure that Gabe did not need any more medical attention.

Everyone was very excited to go home.

"Mummy!" Angel called. "I helped Daddy set up Gabe's rocking chair last night. I even tested it out and I know he's going to love it!" She beamed with pride.

"I know he will. Thanks love. You are the best big sister ever!" Jane smiled, marveling at how mature her two-year-old daughter was acting.

As predicted, Gabe loved his rocking chair.

Every two hours, he woke like clockwork to be fed, burped and rocked back to sleep. He had a very healthy appetite. He paid a visit to his Pediatrician a few days after he was discharged. The Doctor noted that he no longer looked jaundiced. Jane and Jide were very relieved.

The Pediatrician informed them that the results from Gabe's newborn screening test was still pending.

Chapter Six

The Results

Jide came into the bedroom where Jane was feeding the ravenous little Gabe. The grave expression on his face alarmed Jane.

"Why do you look so worried?" She asked him.

"The pediatrician's office called." Jide stated.

Her heartbeat increased, she heard a buzzing sound in her ears and her vision deemed. She held her breath waiting for him to continue. He said nothing more.

"What did they want?" She prompted.

"Gabe has sickle cell disease;" he whispered.

Jane instantly place her hands over Gabe's ears.

She stared at Jide in disbelief.

"Are they sure? Could the results be wrong?" She asked her voice tight with varying emotions.

"They said that the test will be repeated by his hematologist. But the results most likely will remain the same. The results showed only two kinds of hemoglobin. Hemoglobin S; sickle shaped red blood cells, and hemoglobin F; fetal hemoglobin. There was no hemoglobin A." Jide explained.

"We should receive an official letter in the mail very soon." Jide continued. "What we have to do now is find a hematologist and make an appointment."

Jane felt like her world was crumbling. Tears flooded her eyes and flowed down her cheeks. Her nightmare, had just become a reality.

Looking down at the face of her son, she began to visualize him without sickle cell disease.

As shocking as the diagnosis was, it was not unexpected. They had discussed the possibility years before and made plans for this day. Secretly, they both prayed that this day would never come.

Jide shifted uncomfortably at the door. Jane's tears always made him feel uneasy.

"Stop crying." He said. "We made preparations for this day, everything will be ok."

"Let's focus our energy on choosing a good hematologist. Once we make an appointment, we will inform the doctor that we saved Angel's umbilical cord blood. We'll let them know that we want it tested, as soon as possible for compatibility. "Mark my words, he won't have the disease for long," Jide spoke with great conviction.

"Ok." wept Jane.

Chapter Seven

Love defies Logic

Jane was a registered pharmacist and Jide a registered nurse when they met. Why did they choose to get married?

Were they not aware that they both carried the sickle cell trait? Hmmm...

Born in Michigan to Nigerian parents, Jane spent thirteen years of her childhood in Nigeria. Growing up in Nigeria, Jane was very conversant with the ups and downs associated with sickle cell disease (SCD). She lost a barely four-year-old relative to an infection stemming from the complications of sickle cell disease. She also had a friend who frequently battled with sickle cell crisis and fatigue. These experiences gave her an insight on how debilitating SCD can be.

Most people are familiar with the pains associated with SCD, but they do not know the etiology of the disease. Due to the high incidence of malaria in Nigeria, the general population can pay for a test at the doctor's office, to ascertain their genotype.

Many fear the disease, and forbid family members from marrying individuals afflicted with SCD. It was an unwritten rule in Jane's community, that anyone with sickle cell trait, should never marry another trait carrier. This plan was to help eliminate the chances of giving birth to a baby with SCD.

Jane could easily recall instances, where relatives with sickle cell trait, ended major relationships, just because they discovered that their partner, also carried the trait.

In Nigeria, children born with sickle cell disease were unpredictably sickly and were not expected to live a very long life. Jane made up her mind in her teenage years, that she would never marry anyone who carried the sickle cell trait, like she did.

Jide on the other hand, was born in Brooklyn, New York. His mother was Nigerian and his father African-American. Although Jide was identified at birth as a sickle cell trait carrier, he was not counseled about the significance of the gene as a young adult.

Growing up, he did not have any close friends with sickle cell disease. He did not grow up thinking; he would never marry a girl with sickle cell trait.

Chapter Eight

Jide Meets Jane

On a cold autumn afternoon, Jane; a pharmacy intern, had an appointment with the employee health department in a local hospital. She needed to submit a urine sample for drug testing. When she got to the office, she was greeted and directed to the restroom.

"The specimen bags are on the table outside the restroom," the nurse informed her.

When Jane got to the table, she noticed that the bags had the month and day of birth printed boldly on them.

She quickly located her date of birth and grabbed the bag. Entering the restroom, she got ready to make the necessary deposit, but something was not quite right. The date of birth was right but the name was wrong. She readjusted herself, washed her hands and headed out to the table again. Upon closer inspection, she located her bag.

"I wonder who this person is with a Nigerian first name and my date of birth." Jane pondered. "Maybe we will meet on this job and become friends!"

"We already have two things in common; our birthday and Nigerian heritage."

Jane was a hopeless romantic. The incident played in her head all day.

"What are the odds?" She rehashed the story with her roommate that night.

"We must also think alike." She continued, "to look for a new job around the same time, get hired and schedule our screening test for the same day!"

"It must be a match made in heaven," her roommate teased.

"I cannot wait to meet him." Jane said dreamily.

Four months later, they met! Their love story is one for another book.

Chapter Nine

Wedding Bells

Five years later, their love waxed strong. Fueled by their shared love for sports, travel, children and so much more, they decided to get married. At the onset of their relationship, Jane made it clear to Jide, that she would never marry anyone who carried the sickle cell trait. He assured her that there was nothing to worry about since he, did not carry the trait.

One cold winter evening, Jane's close friend; Lara called. Her three years old son; Micheal, was diagnosed with sickle cell disease at birth and most of his three short years were spent going in and out of the hospital. He had frequent sickle cell crisis.

"I've used up all my allocated sick days for the year and it's only March! I can't make plans for vacations, because I'm afraid we won't be able to make it. My husband and I can't figure out what his triggers are! Every aspect of my life is unstable right now." She cried.

She was a night nurse in a large and demanding hospital.

"I need to find a job setting that is accommodating." She paused. A pregnant silence followed.

"My family depends on my salary as you know. I can't afford to lose my job." She continued.

"I love my son so much. I hate that he is suffering like this. I find myself feeling helpless when he's in so much pain." She sobbed.

They both sobbed quietly for a few minutes. Jane did not know how to console her friend, but she had to say something.

"I know this is very challenging;" She began, "somehow, this is bound to get better, Lara. Remember, science is always evolving. I will pray that researchers, come up with a cure very soon."

"I truly pray so." Lara agreed. "Let's talk about something less emotional."

When the phone call ended, Jane was emotionally shaken. She thought about Jide's answer whenever she asked about his genotype.

Something about it, did not sound definite. She found him in his game room, playing a video game.

Pretending that it was not such a serious issue, she asked him yet again.

"Jide, what is your genotype?"

"I am not too sure; he answered breezily. I may have sickle cell trait." He looked at Jane apologetically.

"What!" Jane exclaimed; horrified. "Is this definite?"

"I checked with my mother and she confirmed. I do carry the trait."

Jane could not believe what she was hearing. She was devastated.

"When were you going to tell me?" She demanded.

With over five years invested in this truly loving relationship, she did not know what to do.

Jide felt like a load had been lifted off his shoulders. Initially, when Jane asked him a few years ago, he was sure he had nothing to worry about. However, he decided to confirm with his mother. Her response shocked him. Since then, he was waiting for the perfect opportunity to break the news to Jane.

"This is not the end of the world Jane." He reasoned, "people go through struggles in their relationship, this may be our test."

Jane felt betrayed. She started to withdraw emotionally from Jide.

"How could he not know that he has the trait?" She questioned.

"He is fully aware that marrying someone with sickle cell trait, is not my preference!"

For two weeks, she avoided Jide.

Chapter Ten

Death of a Sister

Two weeks later, Jane received a phone call from her eldest sister Grace.

Grace sensed the turmoil that Jane was going through.

"Is everything okay with you and Jide? Does he anticipate and meet your needs?" Grace asked lovingly.

"Well, I don't have too much needs. You know how independent I am." Jane explained. "Jide is very caring and supportive."

How do I bring up this sickle cell trait issue? Jane wondered.

Deciding to table the discussion for another time, she changed the topic.

Grace recently gave birth to her second son; Daniel.

The last time they spoke, Grace complained of rapid weight loss, night sweat and fatigue.

"How are you doing, Grace? How is Danny feeding?"

Jane asked

"Danny eats almost every hour." Grace tiredly responded.

"This nephew of yours, is very greedy." She joked.

Jane could see her shaking her head. It had been two years since she last saw her eldest sister and she missed her terribly. Jane planned go see her in a few months. She could not wait to meet her nephews.

"You sound tired Grace. More tired than usual. Are you not getting any rest?" Jane was getting alarmed by her sister's energy level. Grace was usually very bubbly.

"I'm not sure what's happening." Grace confided, "I am still having night sweats, I feel extremely weak, I don't have much appetite and I have lost more than the pregnancy weight."

"Have you gone to the hospital?" Jane asked. Trying to think of what could possibly be the cause of these symptoms.

"Don't worry big sister, I will send you some great prenatal vitamins to give you energy." Jane promised. She made a mental note to send the vitamins to Grace, the next day.

A few weeks later, Grace developed orbital cellulites, it alarmed everyone in the family. Grace was the eldest of six girls and all her sisters admired and respected her. She was a strong and healthy independent woman. She always put the needs of her family ahead of everything. Ebby her first son was barely three years old. Everyone was relieved when the orbital cellulites responded to treatment, and resolved.

The next time Jane called Grace, she joked about the scar around her eye.

"Don't worry about that." Jane assured her.

"Once you visit me in New York, we will find you an excellent dermatologist. They will do wonders for you. We're all just thankful that you have recovered."

"I still don't feel like myself." Grace admitted. "I think it's time to go to the hospital for more tests."

A few days later Grace called.

"The result is out," she said. "It is leukemia."

Jane was dumbfounded.

The shocking news rocked to the entire family. Grace had just given birth to a healthy baby boy, she had no previous medical issues and her baby was barely three months old. How could this be happening?

Jane quickly pulled out her textbooks and read all she could about the disease. She had currently met a patient who survived a type of leukemia. She prayed that Grace would have the same results.

The leukemia was acute and aggressive. She was diagnosed with acute lymphoblastic leukemia. Grace lived in Nigeria with her family. The medical plan was for her to become stabilized enough to travel to the Unites States of America for medical treatment. Surely, one of her five siblings would be a match for a bone marrow transplant. Stabilization proved elusive. One day Grace was full of energy and the next, she needed emergency blood transfusion.

Medications for treatment were not readily available at the teaching hospital, where she was admitted. Prescribed medications had to be purchased by the family, from all over the country. How could a hospital have a treatment protocol, without medications? Despite the drawbacks, everyone remained optimistic.

Barely three months after diagnosis Grace died. She was only thirty-five years old.

The months that followed was like a nightmare.

Grief came with so much anger, as Jane mourned her sister. She reanalyzed every aspect of her life. Life was truly too short; Jane decided.

Slowly, she opened up her heart to Jide once again.

Together Jane and Jide started to research the advancements made in the sickle cell disease world. They decided that they would use gene selection when the time came to have their children. They would also save each baby's umbilical cord blood to have as a health insurance.

Less than five months after, Jide proposed marriage to Jane and she accepted. They began to plan their wedding. Jane did not tell her parents about the sickle cell trait issue. She knew they would discourage her.

Chapter Eleven

The Right Hematologist

The pediatrician's office recommended two hematologists on Staten Island; where they lived. They read numerous patient reviews and called the doctor's offices to asked numerous questions. They wanted to make sure that the selected specialist, had at least one practice site, in an area with a dense population of sickle cell disease patients.

They decided on the hematologist, whose office was close to their home. The doctor was very involved in the sickle cell community, and was affiliated with a hospital in Brooklyn; an area in New York City that has a good population of sickle cell disease patients.

Although sickle cell disease affects people of different races, it is more prominent in people of African descent. About one in three hundred and sixty-five African Americans have the disease.

So why did Jane and Jide put so much effort into finding the right doctor?

You will understand their reasoning, once you become familiar with the disease.

Chapter Twelve

Sickle Cell Disease

A long time ago in the tropics, many people died from malaria; a disease transmitted by bites from female anopheles mosquitoes infected with a parasite called plasmodium. Malaria is characterized by symptoms such as fever and chills, headaches, seizures, convulsions, diarrhea, nausea and vomiting, anemia, jaundice, muscle pain and rectal bleeding.

In its divine awesomeness, the human body made a vital change to its genes also known as; genetic mutation. Some of the red blood cells changed shape.

Yes, this is the time to pull out that dictionary!

Due to this genetic mutation, red blood cells in the body, which are normally shaped like disc and are very flexible, became sickled and rigid. This mutation is believed to have improved malaria survival rate.

People with the sickle cell trait have thirty-five percent or less sickle cells circulating in their blood stream at any given time. As time went on, people with the trait started to intermarry. Once they started having children, they noticed that one or more of their offspring would get sick very often or die young.

Scientists discovered that when both parents have the sickle cell trait, with any given pregnancy, there is a twenty-five percent chance that the child would be born with sickle cell disease.

Why? You may ask?

Well, each parent with the sickle cell trait has one regular cell and one sickle cell. When a child is consummated, each parent randomly donates a gene to make up the child's gene. If the gene donated from both mother and father are sickle cells, then the child will be born with sickle cell disease.

Sickle red blood cells have a life span of at most, twenty days in the blood stream, while normal red blood cells have the life span of one hundred and twenty days.

Red blood cells have a protein called hemoglobin. Hemoglobin is in charge of carrying oxygen to all parts of the body. As the blood makes it journey through the body, it passes thorough the spleen for detoxification.

Disc shaped red blood cells due to their flexibility, flow out of the spleen after this process. Sickle cells due to their rigidity and inflexibility get stuck in the filters, clogging up the spleen. With sickle cells trapped in the spleen, fewer red blood cells are left to circulate in the blood stream. This is the main cause of anemia in sickle cell disease patients.

The spleen works very hard to destroy these sickled cells. It breaks down the hemoglobin in the cells which leads to the release of bilirubin; an orange-yellow pigment that builds up in the blood stream, causing jaundice. Jaundice is seen very prominently as yellowing of the white part of the eye; sclera, in patients.

An overworked spleen may start to harden, get inflamed and sometimes, need to be surgically removed. For this reason, parents of babies and young children with sickle cell disease are taught to palpate the spleen. This is basically feeling for a mass or hardening right underneath the ribcage on the left side of the chest.

Although one can live without their spleen, they are losing one component of their body, that helps fight infections.

Sickle cells love to clog up small vessels in the body. They can do this at any time and without warning. If they clog up small vessels in the brain; it can lead to a stroke. In males, they can clog up small vessels in the penis causing painful prolonged erections; priapism. Prolonged periods of priapism can ultimately lead to impotence. Sickle cells can clog up small blood vessels in the lungs, causing extreme pain; Acute Chest Syndrome. In babies, sickle cells can clog up small vessels in hands and feet, causing swelling and pain.

Uneventful clogs can eventually lead to ulcers, bone pain, all kinds of infections, eye damages, and more.

Sickle cell disease is characterized with sudden onset of acute pain, chronic pain, chronic anemia, depression and more.

Presently, patients are treated both prophylactically and symptomatically. Blood work is done as often as necessary to monitor hemoglobin levels and the functions of the kidney and liver.

Brain scan is done irregularly to make sure that patients have not had minor clots in their brain. There is also a cure. It is not an easy treatment. However, it is worth considering, if the opportunity presents itself. Due to the fact that the disease progression is different in every patient, picking a knowledgeable hematologist is the most important step in managing and overcoming this disease.

Chapter Thirteen

Visiting the Hematologist

The hematologist; Dr. Pee is a kind and knowledgeable doctor. He is very involved in the sickle cell disease community and actively networks with other specialists in and out of his field. There was something comforting about being in his office.

Jane and Jide went to all of Gabe's appointments as a family unit. During their first visit, Jide informed Dr. Pee, that Angel's cord blood was in storage for Gabe's treatment.

"How did you know to save your daughter's cord blood?" Dr. Pee asked.

"Well;" Jide responded, "once we found out that we both carried the sickle cell trait, we explored options available to have a healthy baby."

"Our initial plan was to do gene selection;" Jide continued, meaning his sperm was to be collected at a lab, analyzed to isolate sperms without the sickle cell gene. Jane will then receive the sperm via artificial insemination.

This is a rigorous process that involves monitoring ovulation cycle, and sometimes oral and injectable medications to prepare Jane's body.

"My gynecologist at the time advised against this." Jane interjected. "I had an early miscarriage with an unexpected pregnancy and she did not want me to become extremely anxious about having another baby."

"After thorough research, we decided to take a chance with the first pregnancy, then save the umbilical cord blood. We read that this can be used to cure sickle cell disease." Jane finished.

There are a whole lot of diseases that can be cured using the cord blood and sickle cell disease is one of them.

The patient undergoes a short course of chemotherapy to wipe out their bone marrow, then the stem cells from a compatible donor is infused. The infused cells will adapt to their environment and produce more healthy donor cells. At the end of treatment, the patient will take on the genotype of the donor.

Dr. Pee was very impressed with their preparedness.

"It is too early to think of a transplant now," He advised. "Some children have a mild case of the disease. The best thing to do, is to monitor him closely and see how the disease progresses."

In the meantime, Gabe was started on prophylactic penicillin. He took a dose in the morning and another at night.

It is recommended that children born with sickle cell disease, take antibiotics for the first five years of their life. This is to prevent infections, which can trigger a crisis leading to hospitalization and sometimes death. The family embraced this treatment.

Dr. Pee also stressed the importance of hydration and gave further instructions.

"Do not limit Gabe," he cautioned, "allow him to set his own pace when it comes to physical activities."

"Palpate the spleen often;" he continued, showing them how to properly perform this physical examination.

"Any kind of fever is an emergency," he cautioned, "and if he starts crying uncontrollably, watch for any signs that he is guarding his hands or feet; this is also a sign of crisis."

Jane and Jide left the visit feeling both overwhelmed and hopeful. They prayed that Gabe would have the mild form of the disease. If he did not, they took some comfort in the fact that they had another option, to help him overcome the disease.

As they drove home that day, they were thankful that they picked a knowledgeable and caring doctor.

Chapter Fourteen

The Medical Plan

Two years prior to Gabe's birth, Angel's umbilical cord blood was collected from the delivery room for storage. A few weeks later, the pediatrician's office called Jane and her husband.

"The newborn screening test results are in. Angel carries the sickle cell trait." The doctor informed them.

They were relieved. Angel did not have sickle cell disease. For Jane and Jide, the stored cord blood became a symbol of hope. The pediatrician instructed them to make sure Angel was adequately hydrated.

"Be sure to limit physical activity at high altitude or in extreme temperatures." The doctor continued.

Individuals with sickle cell trait can become symptomatic in these settings. This is especially true in competitive sports.

"Make sure that Angel eats a balanced diet and gets plenty of rest." The doctor concluded.

Jane and Jide resolved to adhere to the doctor's counseling.

Chapter Fifteen

One Year Later

Twice a year, the entire family made the trip to the hematologist's office; to see Dr. Pee. The children look forward to getting stickers and candy at the end of the visit. All Jane and Jide wanted, was confirmation that Gabe was thriving. With every visit, they had one thought in mind; Will this be the visit that would activate the medical plan?

Thankfully, Gabe's first year was uneventful. His parents did everything they could, to maintain a healthy home. Angel and Gabe stayed home with either their parents or grandparents. This was done to avoid daycare related germs; children recycle too many viruses and bacteria.

As Gabe grew, so did his appetite. He loved to drink water and milk. He loved his fruits, vegetables and even his penicillin. He also had a lot of energy, barely crawling before he started to walk and climb. Like most younger siblings do, he followed Angel around, like her shadow.

His fetal hemoglobin stayed highly elevated, above twenty-five percent. This is the hemoglobin that carries oxygen from a mother to her fetus, in the last seven months of development. In most cases, it declines quickly after birth and by the second birthday, there is barely any circulating in the blood stream. One of the ways to treat sickle cell disease is to give patients a medication; Hydroxyurea, it reactivates the production of fetal hemoglobin. Fetal hemoglobin has the highest affinity for oxygen.

Dr. Pee was amazed.

"Does anyone in your family have a history of elevated fetal hemoglobin?" He asked.

Neither Jane nor Jide had any idea. However, they were very happy to get this news.

"Do you think we could be so lucky and Gabe's fetal hemoglobin will stay elevated forever?" Ever the optimist, Jane asked excitedly.

"Maybe Gabe will not have to undergo the stem cell transplant after all!" She said wistfully.

"We will continue to monitor him. As long he has no complications, we don't have to worry about testing for compatibility with the stem cells, just yet." counseled Dr. Pee.

"The test requires a large volume of blood from both of your children." He added.

Chapter Sixteen

Emergency Room Visit

Like the first year, the second year was also medically uneventful for Gabe. However, he made a trip to the emergency room for a non-sickle cell disease related event. It happened one autumn afternoon, while Jane was at work at the pharmacy.

"How is your son doing?" Her current patient asked.

Most of the patients at the pharmacy knew her, during her pregnancy. They loved to inquire about Gabe, every time they visited the pharmacy.

"Oh, he's doing great! He's standing and pulling every…" Jane was interrupted midsentence when one of her technicians; Dominique, called her name.

"Sounds like your husband on the phone." Dominique said.

"I'll be right back." Jane excused herself, hurrying to answer the phone. Jide was currently in graduate school. He never calls at this time of the day; she thought.

"Hello?" She answered.

"Rush back to my parents' house immediately!" Jide sounded frantic.

"Gabe has had an acid…."

Jane felt lifeless. Her skin felt like it was just doused with a bucket of ice water.

Jide's voice faded in and out of her ear.

She heard the words "burn", "screaming" and dropped the phone. Tears rolled down her cheeks.

She heard a wailing sound and was surprised when people came to console her.

She was not sure what was wrong.

"You can't do anything under these conditions;" her patient said, "I'll take you to where you need to go."

The fifteen-minutes ride to her In-law's house felt like an eternity.

"Don't worry, everything will work out just fine." Consoled Ms. Kay; her patient turned good Samaritan.

She tried to console Jane by telling her stories of family members who got into serious scraps as children.

"James my cousin's son even had the hot oil accident." Mrs. Kay continued.

"It was so terrible but he survived it."

"You would think he would learn from such an accident. He later died from gang related issues when he was much older…"

At this point, Jane tuned her out. Praying silently as they drove along in slow-moving traffic.

"God, I know you will never put more on me, than I can bear. Please heal him even as I pray. Amen." She kept repeating this prayer over and over to draw strength.

Finally, the car turned into the familiar tree lined street. The usually serene street felt eerie. Hurriedly expressing her gratitude to Mrs. Kay, Jane sprinted towards the unusually quiet house.

She met a sad looking Grandpa at the door.

"Where is Gabe?" She asked.

"In the bedroom." A contrite Grandpa responded.

Running to the bedroom, she found Gabe fast asleep. A quick survey of his face, showed that he did not have any facial injuries. Jane breathed a prayer of thanks. Peeling back his onesie, she noted that he had sustained burns on the skin covering his left clavicle. It looked terrible and gave Jane instant goosebumps.

"He pulled down a hot cup of tea from the kitchen table." She heard Grandpa explain somewhere behind her.

"Just a week ago, he could barely reach that table." Grandpa said perplexed.

Heart racing and silent tears running down her cheeks, she carried Gabe out of the house and headed towards the car, which was parked in the drive way. Grandpa quietly followed with Angel in tow. The usually chatty Angel was silent. She witnessed her brother's accident and listened to him cry till he fell asleep. They silently drove to the local pediatric emergency room.

At the emergency room, vital signs showed that Gabe was in stable condition. The usual emergency room delay followed. Sitting in an allocated room, Jane began to worry that he would get an infection. The wound was yet to be cleaned, despite the fact that Jane informed the nurse, that Gabe had sickle cell disease.

The medical resident was more interested in finding out whether this was a case of child abuse. Jane was emotionally and physically drained.

Gabe had woken up and was unusually quiet. He quietly stared at Jane. Jane called her younger sister Sally to tell her of the incident. Once Sally picked up her phone, Jane found that she could not get any words out. She started sobbing uncontrollably. The phone reception was very poor and the phone disconnected.

The medical resident came in; for the fourth time.

"Where was this tea that he pulled down?" He asked again.

Jane became angry, before she could respond, Jide arrived.

He had driven from Pennsylvania to Brooklyn in record time.

"What is happening here?" Jide demanded.

"Why has my son not been seen, treated and discharged?"

"There is no one here. This Emergency room is basically empty!" He fired questions at the medical resident.

"I have a few questions to ask," the resident began but was cut off by Jide.

"Did you not write down the answers to these questions? You asked my wife these same questions almost an hour ago!" Jide was in rare form.

"This is a sickle cell disease patient. I hope you know what that means. He cannot be here for much longer. His presence here, increases his risk of infections." Jide was infuriated.

"Kindly get me the attending physician, since you cannot take care of this situation on your own."

Few minutes later, the attending physician arrived. She looked overworked, stated that it was only a minor burn and began treatment. She wiped the wound clean with Betadine; Gabe broke his silence then, screaming in pain. She wrote prescriptions for a burn cream and a new antibiotic. Gabe was to stop taking his routine penicillin; until he completed the new antibiotic regimen. He was discharged. A couple of weeks later, the burn healed leaving behind a little discoloration.

Chapter Seventeen

Vacations

Every summer, the family went on vacation to a location in the Caribbean Islands for a week or two. Gabe had no qualms wading in the shallow shores of the ocean. His parents made sure to only visit the beach in the afternoon, after the hot sun had adequately warmed the turquoise colored ocean.

Slathered in sun screen, Gabe would engage in all kinds of water games and build sand castles.

Jane and Jide ensured that the surrounding outdoor swimming pool was also warm.

You may recall that extreme heat or cold temperatures, serve as triggers for sickle cell crisis; warm temperature is preferred.

Chapter Eighteen

Yellow Eyes and Fatigue

After his third birthday, Gabe experienced a growth spurt. He was much taller and added a healthy weight; thanks to his great appetite and physical activity.

However, Jane noticed that his sclera; the white part of the eye was not as white as his sister's.

She also noticed that he started taking long naps, especially after periods of play. He was currently on two medications at this time; the prophylactic penicillin and folic acid.

Based on the result from his current blood work, his hemoglobin level was now nine grams per deciliter. The normal range for a male child is between eleven to thirteen grams per deciliter. He had previously had a level of ten grams per deciliter. Jane and Jide began to discuss the use of the cord blood again.

During his scheduled visit to Dr. Pee, the doctor began to discuss the initiation of Hydroxyurea; a medication used to increase fetal hemoglobin in patients with sickle cell disease. Some patients on this medication achieve up to twenty percent or more increase in their fetal hemoglobin levels. Jane and Jide declined starting the medication. However, they took the prescription home. They resolved to test the cord blood first and if Gabe could not use it, then they would initiate hydroxyurea.

They made an appointment and took both of their children to a nearby hospital for the necessary blood work. The day of the blood draw was intense. There were lots of test tubes to collect blood samples. Angel took a look at the test tubes and started wailing. She noticed that her name was on one of the forms. She realized that she was also there for a blood draw.

After the blood draw, Jane and Jide left the hospital with tears in their eyes. They had an overwhelming feeling that they were about to embark on a challenging journey.

"God, please give me the strength needed for this next chapter of our lives." Jane prayed.

"At least the blood work is finally completed," said Jide. "Let's hope for the best."

Chapter Nineteen

Test Results

At the next visit, Dr. Pee was overjoyed to share with Jane and her husband the results from the blood tests. Angel and Gabe were one hundred percent match! It was a dream come true. Dr. Pee immediately gave them the contact information for a transplant doctor in a renowned children's hospital.

Excited and emboldened by the results, Jane immediately made an appointment to meet with the transplant doctor, on their way home. Gabe's journey to overcome sickle cell disease had just begun.

The transplant doctor and nurse practitioner at the hospital were very pleasant. They exuded an aura of genuine care, and gave the impression that they truly loved their job. They explained the entire transplant process to Gabe's parents. The transplant program at Morgan Stanley Children's Hospital; one of the highly ranked children's hospitals, had over ninety percent success rate, in sibling to sibling bone marrow transplant.

Jane and her husband left their first appointment feeling very overwhelmed. They were handed a huge binder that outlined the entire transplant process. They also received contact information for a parent, whose child had undergone the same process, five years prior.

To begin the treatment, Gabe had to meet the study criteria. First, he had to undergo a series of pre-transplant tests. This consisted of an extensive blood work, organ scans, as well as a physical and psychological examination.

These tests were to obtain a baseline on the effects of sickle cell disease on his body. The results from the test, would also help determine if Gabe's major organs, could handle the chemotherapeutic part of treatment. If the results come back within an acceptable range, treatment will begin.

It was going to take about six months for Gabe to achieve a cure. One week of chemotherapy, four to six weeks stay in the hospital and about twelve weeks spent at home; recuperating.

Chapter Twenty

Pre-transplant Testing

One of the pre-transplant procedures that made Gabe's parents anxious, was the Magnetic Resonance Imaging (MRI). Recent result from Gabe's blood work, showed that his hemoglobin level had declined further from ten to seven grams per deciliter. In order for Gabe to undergo the MRI, his hemoglobin level had to be at least ten grams per deciliter, as per hospital protocol. Gabe was going to receive his first blood transfusion a week or so before the procedure.

Gabe's parents were distressed. They worried about Gabe's declining hemoglobin levels. They prayed that he would not have any transfusion reaction. They were aware that general anesthesia caused sickling in sickle cell disease patients, and Gabe had to receive anesthesia for the MRI. Despite these concerns; they believed that they were on the right path. They trusted the hospital's protocol and the transplant team explicitly.

Jane and Jide deliberated. "It is better for Gabe to receive this transplant, as soon as possible." Jane concluded, "He will forget all about it in a few years."

To deal with her anxiety, Jane formulated a daily prayer. *"Dear God, I believe that we are on the right path. It may not be a smooth path, but I know it will end well. I believe that this treatment is already successful. Amen."*

Chapter Twenty-one

Gabe asks Questions

Gabe was a very inquisitive and intelligent little boy.

His parents never mentioned to him that he was sick. Recently, he noticed that he was frequenting the hospital and doing all kinds of tests.

He also overheard the nurse practitioner inform his parents that he needed a blood transfusion.

"What is a blood transfusion and why am I getting it?" Gabe asked Jane.

Jane did not want to scare Gabe. She thought of the best way to break the news.

At almost four years old, Gabe was in love with teenage mutant ninja turtles. He was constantly talking about defeating Shredder and his gang of bad guys.

"There are some bad guys in your blood and this blood transfusion is to help you fight and defeat them." Jane smiled.

Gabe was happy with this answer.

"Where is the blood coming from?" Gabe asked; after a few minutes.

"The blood bank," Jane responded swallowing the sudden lump in her throat.

"Let's see if we can spot the delivery from the blood bank when it arrives Gabe." Jane exclaimed suddenly.

She felt the need to keep Gabe excited about the procedure.

A smile formed on Gabe's lips and his light-yellow eyes lit up.

"Who is from the blood bank?" He asked no one in particular.

"Is he from the blood bank, Mummy?" He pointed at a toddler riding a toy wagon.

"That baby cannot be from the blood bank!" Jane laughed

Soon they were both laughing. The game eased all tension.

"Mummy! I see the blood." Gabe pointed

There it was indeed!

His nurse received the blood and confirmed that it was for him. The transfusion began shortly after. Thankfully, the transfusion was uneventful. He was observed for an hour and sent home. Gabe fell asleep on the way home. He slept for hours.

A few days after the blood transfusion, Jane noted that his sclera; the white part of his eyes was milky white again and his energy level had doubled.

"We are making the right decision," she muttered to herself.

Chapter Twenty-two

Just Enough Cord Blood

The cord blood was delivered to the hospital by the storage company for analysis and preparation. During this process, the transplant team calculated how much volume they would need for the procedure. They realized that the actual volume was just enough to perform the transplant.

"We will prefer to have a little more than Gabe needs, just in case he needs to undergo this treatment twice," the transplant doctor said to Jane and Jide, in her usual caring manner.

Since the transplant date was a few weeks away, they worried that like most children do, Gabe will have a little more growth.

Jane and Jide had to decide on the next alternative. Getting fresh bone marrow from their daughter; Angel. She would have to undergo some tests to make sure that she was healthy enough to donate. In a twinkle of an eye, the medical plan was switching from a stem cell transplant to a bone marrow transplant.

They truly did not want to have both of their children undergo major medical procedures at the same time. But what could they do? They could not allow Gabe to go through a week of grueling chemotherapy and not have sufficient bone marrow to help cure the disease.

The decision though very difficult, was made.

Chapter Twenty-three

Jane calls Nigerian Aunty Cecilia

It was now in five-year-old Angel's hands to give her consent. She could not be forced to make this donation.

Now this idea, is a novelty! Anyone raised in a Nigerian home understands that parents make all major decisions in the household. A child under sixteen years of age, definitely had no say.

Even though Jane was born in American, she spent the formative years of her life in Nigeria. The Nigerian in Jane, worried that her very outspoken daughter would get scared and refuse the procedure. She had not even told Angel the reason why, they suddenly had to go to the hospital so often.

Jane could still remember the last time her children asked her about the numerous blood work Gabe had to undergo.

"Mummy, why do we have to go to the clinic so much?" Angel once asked.

"Well, Gabe has some bad guys in his blood that have to be defeated." Jane started, praying that Angel would not demand more explanation.

"If they are not defeated, they could make him very sick at any time." She finished.

"We don't want that to happen." Angel said in her usual thoughtful way.

"Gabe, don't worry;" Angel assured her brother, "we will all make sure that all the bad guys are destroyed!".

There was no doubt, Angel truly loved her little brother.

Jane did not want to unnerve Angel by telling her about the bone marrow harvest procedure. She decided to call her favorite Aunt; Cecilia, to clear her head and calm her nerves.

Aunty Cecilia; like she was fondly called, was a no non-sense Nigerian woman. She was not a blood relative. However, in Nigeria, anyone older than you by as little as one day can be referred to as Aunty or Uncle; if they demand it.

Aunty Cecilia was single and in her late forties. She was once engaged to be married and had a terrible heartbreak. She had weathered that storm in her life and emerged from it, a warrior. A self-appointed authority in all matters of the heart, she was fun, generous, a straight shooter and Jane loved her.

"Aunty Cecilia?" Jane asked, as soon as someone picked up the phone on the other end.

"Who else will it be, abi no be me you call?" Aunty Cecilia joked.

She had a way of dropping her polished Nigerian-American accent and speaking in broken English.

"We don enter oo." Jane said in a quiet emotional voice

"Wetin happen now?" Aunty Cecilia asked.

"They talk say Angel must give consent for them to get bone marrow from her."

"Ah Ah?!" Aunty Cecilia exclaimed.

"What does a child know about these things? Anyway, it will be ok. The Angel I know will say yes."

"Meanwhile, if you had not married Jide when you found out that he carried the sickle cell trait, all these things would have been avoided." She chided in her usual pragmatic tone.

Jane rolled her eyes.

"Here we go again," she mumbled under her breath.

"Do you know how many tall, handsome well-to-do men I turned down for this same reason. Ehh?"

Jane grimaced, it was time to get off the phone.

"Aunty please," she huffed. "Just keep praying for us abeg."

"Meanwhile, let me call you back please. The hospital is calling again." Jane fibbed. She had no energy to cry over spilt milk. This was not the time to analyze her marriage to Jide.

"Ok o, we go continue later." Aunty Cecilia agreed, hearing the strain in Jane's voice. "All will be well my dear."

Jane quickly hung up, exhaling loudly. Later that night, she spoke with Jide and they decided not to alarm Angel.

"I think it's best to have a trained professional ask Angel the questions." Jide suggested.

Chapter Twenty-four

Psychological Evaluation

Everyone in the family had to undergo a psychological evaluation. This was to make sure that they were mentally ready for Gabe's treatment. The treatment was sure to bring major changes in the daily activities of the entire family. Jane had to take six months unpaid time-off from work, to be with Gabe in the hospital. For this to happen, Jide could not afford to miss any day from work. His parents, especially his mother; Loveline, would help to make sure that Angel did not feel neglected, while her brother was in the hospital. Loveline, went with Jane for the psychological evaluation appointment.

Jane's relationship with Loveline was great. It used to make Jide jealous in the beginning of their courtship.

"Why do you act like my mother is the match maker that set us up? Jide asked on numerous occasions, what exactly are you guys talking about for so long on the phone?" He queried at other times.

Jane always found this comical.

"Well, your mother and I have a lot in common," Jane responded carefully.

"We both love Nigerian food and we speak a common second language; Igbo. There is also gardening and family events, to discuss! Just be happy we get along marvelously." Jane gave him a dimpled smile.

Loveline and her husband Larry spent a lot of time with their only grandchildren; Angel and Gabe. Due to Gabe's treatment, Angel was going to spend even more time with her grandparents. Jane knew that Angel would definitely be coddled by her grandparents.

Angel's encounter with the psychologist was refreshing and encouraging.

"Angel; did you know that your brother had sickle cell disease?" The friendly psychologist asked.

Angel tilted her head to the side and puckered her mouth; she was processing this new information.

A pregnant silence followed.

"He will need some help from you." The psychologist resumed the conversation.

Angel's head shot up and she looked at Jane for a brief second. Jane could see the question in Angel's eyes; is this the truth?

Jane nodded her head.

"What kind of help does Gabe need?" Angel asked.

"We would need some bone marrow from you, so that he can have a chance to live a healthy life."

"I will do anything for my brother," Angel said smiling. She sat back on her chair, squared her shoulders and lifted her head high. She was proud to be of help.

Jane felt her throat tighten, and just like that, the anxiety surrounding the entire appointment faded away.

Jane could not wait to tell Jide the good news.

Later on, she was informed by the transplant team, that the bone marrow harvest would take place the day following Gabe's hospital admission.

Chapter Twenty-five

Jide's Motorcycle Accident

Two weeks before Gabe's hospital admission, Jide was involved in a motorcycle accident on his way back from work. He was knocked off his motorcycle, in a head-on collision with a car.

Jide was lucky to emerge from the accident, with only a few rips in his jeans and severe road burn on his buttock, palms, knees and elbows.

In typical macho fashion, he turned down the offer to go to the hospital in the ambulance, claiming he was feeling "just fine." Nothing acts like a natural pain killer better than adrenaline rush. "I'll have my friend drive me home instead." He told the emergency medical technician.

Once he settled in for the car ride, the pain kicked in. Jide arrived home, barely able to walk.

Jane heard the storm door slam and waited for Jide to come up the steps leading into the living room, like he usually does. A few minutes passed and still no Jide. Jane sensed something was wrong. She called out to him His tone sounded strange, when he responded. Deciding to go downstairs to check on him. Nothing prepared her for what she saw.

Jide was hunched over the pool table, his hands were clenched and bleeding, his pants were torn in multiple areas. He looked like someone who just took a hard tumble on granite.

"What happened?" Jane asked very alarmed.

"Can you drive me to the hospital?' Jide whispered grimacing.

"Who brought you home?" She demanded.

"My friend did." Jide answered, grinding his teeth.

"Why couldn't he take you to the nearest hospital? Actually, don't answer that. Let's go." Jane ordered.

Jane ran up the staircase, taking two steps at a time.

She got to the living room out of breath. Her father; D, was sitting and watching family feud with the children.

"I have to take Jide to the hospital, now." Jane grabbed her car keys.

"I should be back in an hour or so."

"What happened? D asked."

"Jide got into an accident." Jane said in a flat tone.

Looking at his grandchildren, D knew that it was not a good time to ask for details

"I'll tell you about it, when I get back."

Jane ran down the steps and ran towards her car. Jide followed her, limping.

Janet drove calmly towards the closest hospital.

"Drive faster!" Jide muttered, "I'm in so much pain."

"Your friend should have driven you directly to the hospital. Sir!"

Her shock, slowly turned into anger.

"You cannot afford to be this careless." Jane spoke coldly, fighting very hard to control her rage.

"You have a car. No? Why don't you use it? Our son is about to undergo a major-medical procedure! I have more than enough to worry about. Please, do not give me any more stress."

Jane rolled her eyes, clucked her teeth and continued to drive.

Jide knew better. He did not respond.

They drove quietly until they arrived at the emergency room. It was Friday evening; the room was eerily quiet. Jide was quickly triaged.

HIs vital signs were normal and most of his wounds where superficial.

He was soon wheeled into a holding room and the medical resident on duty, was paged. The medical resident happened to be an avid biker. He was more interested in the type of bike that Jide was riding.

As they conversed about power bikes, Jane said her goodbyes and slipped out the room.

"Men!" she sighed in relief.

Once in her car, she thanked God for sparing Jide's life.

Chapter Twenty-six

A Week before Check in

The week leading up to Gabe's admission, was the hardest for everyone. Jane had to say goodbye to her co-workers. Initially, they were alarmed. However, once she assured them that it was to cure her son of sickle cell disease, they all wished her well.

At church, Jane mentioned to one of Gabe's sabbath school teachers, that Gabe would not be around for a little while and explained the reasons why. Immediately, the teacher sprang into action. She rallied some elders together and they held hands and prayed for little Gabe, Angel and the medical team involved.

Jane's sisters called her to give her advice and encouragement.

"Do not show Gabe that you're afraid. Be strong and he will be strong." her sister Sally advised.

"Make sure the hospital room smells like home." Her sister Pat advised.

"Do not hesitate to call us, if you need anything." Her sister's Joyce, Isadore and Gift offered.

Jane felt as mentally ready as one could be, under these circumstances.

"Let me call a parent who has gone through this before." She told Jide.

The transplant team had previously given her a few contact information. This was to help connect Jane and her husband, with parents whose children had previously gone through a bone marrow transplant.

Jane called Mrs. Gray. Her son; Gregory went through the process five years ago. Jane had previously exchanged pleasantries with her via electronic mail. Mrs. Gray was a very pleasant lady and was eager to share her experiences. Her son was also three years old when he had his bone marrow transplant procedure. His donor was his younger brother.

"I'm so nervous;" Jane said, once she got on the phone.

Her voice was shaking from her anxiety and restlessness.

"I need your advice. What should I expect during our stay at the hospital?" She asked.

"It's going to be a very challenging six months for you and your family. Just keep in mind, when the dust settles, you'll be glad you did this." Mrs. Gray reassured her.

"Here are a few things to keep in mind. Gregory was toilet trained before the procedure, but he had to be retrained after the treatment"

Jane cringed. She was so proud of Gabe; who basically toilet trained himself before turning three. Gabe was so proud of his accomplishment. "How would this affect him?" Jane wondered.

She was silently thinking about this, when Mrs. Gray interrupted her thoughts.

"It was not for defecation." Mrs. Gray continued, "Gregory was receiving so much intravenously medications and hydrating fluids, that he could not control his bladder, especially at night. His nurse also had to record his fluid intake and urine output. It became more convenient to wear a diaper. This way I didn't have to worry about how much urine was lost on soaked bedsheets."

"I will just take it one step at a time;" Jane muttered to herself.

Mrs. Gray continued; "The bulk of the time spent in the hospital, is actually spent waiting for the body to accept the bone marrow and start making its own cells. Be sure to pack some entertainment for yourself."

Jane did not think she would be in the frame of mind to look for entertainment. She decided to pack a journal instead. She would also bring along the heavy treatment binder that she received at the transplant clinic.

"Don't worry so much about Gabe's entertainment, the child life department at the hospital is excellent;" continued Mrs. Gray, "They'll fill Gabe's day with lots of toys and activities. They even have volunteers to play with him and a school teacher. He will have lots of fun there and soon, he'll forget the entire experience."

"Your job is to keep an eye on Gabe's physical progress. The transplant team responds very quickly to any changes in your child's condition. All you have to do is make them aware, immediately. Since you'll be with him at all times, you will be the first to notice subtle changes."

Jane thanked Mrs. Gray. Now she had a better idea on what to expect.

Later that night, she discussed with Jide and they both agreed that this was another confirmation that they were on the right path.

"God, I know that you have already done it all for me," Jane prayed. "I believe that we are on the right path. It may not be a smooth path but I know it will end well. I believe that this treatment is successful, Amen."

With this prayer, Jane felt calm.

Chapter Twenty-seven

Sunday Afternoon Check-in

That Sunday afternoon, the hospital called that a bed was ready for Gabe. He was expected to check-in that evening, around four. Everyone in the immediate family, drove to the hospital. Angel was scheduled to have a bone marrow harvest the very next day. The transplant team told the parents, that it was alright for Angel to sleep over in Gabe's room that night. This would make Gabe's transition to a hospital room easier; since they shared a room at home. The hospital room was a private room with one bed, a full-sized sofa bed, a desk and chair. It had a toilet and bathroom as well.

Gabe was going to get a central line with three branches inserted, early the next morning. The central line will make it easier for Gabe to receive chemotherapy, blood products, intravenous fluids and other necessary treatments. Gabe's pre-transplant intravenous medications started that night. His penicillin and folic acid where converted from tablets to intravenous medications. Jane sat down and observed her son, he did not look nervous. He had both of his parents and his sister in his room.

The next day, both procedures were successful. Angel was sedated and bone marrow was harvested from her hips. Gabe on the other hand, was sedated and the central line was inserted directly into his heart. With both children in the operating room, Jane was a nervous wreck.

Later that evening, a groggy Angel lounged on the sofa in Gabe's room. Gabe had lots of intravenous lines attached to him. All his medications were attached to a moving rod. Jane looked at both her babies and smiled.

"Things are changing." She whispered to Jide.

Chapter Twenty-eight

Chemotherapy Begins

Chemotherapy started on Gabe's birthday. This was not a coincident. During the planning process, Jane and Jide were both aware that this would happen.

With his transplant team's approval, they took Gabe on an early birthday trip to Saint Marten. They reasoned that he needed some fun memories to sustain him, during his treatment.

To prepare for chemotherapy, Gabe was started on prophylactic medications to help avert dangerous chemotherapy related side effects. Prior to initiating chemotherapy, he received his second blood transfusion. This transfusion like the first, was to prevent crisis. Jane surveyed the nurse's medication table. It was filled with a bunch of emergency medications that Gabe might need during the chemotherapy infusion. She prayed they would not be needed, but she was thankful that they were readily available. Jane took a seat by her son's bed and proceeded to watch him attentively. She did not want to miss any physical changes. Thankfully, there was no noted adverse event.

Later that evening, the nurses and some workers from the child life department, surprised Gabe with a birthday cake. Gabe's room was also decorated with a treatment calendar. This handmade calendar, mapped out his treatment plan from the day of admission, to a predetermined transplant date and finally, a possible discharge date. The calendar was decorated with characters from his favorite television shows; paw patrol and teenage mutant ninja turtle. Everyone sang the happy birthday song, as Gabe happily enjoyed a piece of his cake.

Angel, Jide and his parents, came to visit Gabe later that night.

"What are all these wires connected to Gabe?" Angel asked, somewhat alarmed. She had previously been tired; after her bone marrow harvest procedure, to notice the catheter that was now attached to him.

"That's the best way for Gabe to painlessly get all his medications and that bone marrow you donated!" Jane responded.

"Great! I don't like needles. Neither does Gabe!" Angel responded.

"Don't worry Gabe. Very soon you'll be ready to go home." She added.

Climbing into her brother's bed, they began to watch their television show.

"What's all this beeping sounds, Mummy?" Angel asked. She was referring to the alarm attached to each of Gabe's infusion pumps.

"There are so many different kinds of sounds. It's too noisy!" She lamented holding her ears.

"Those are very important sounds, Angel." Jane explained.

"There is a sound to let us know that the medication is finished, a sound to let us know when Gabe's central line has a kink and the medication cannot enter his body." Jane continued.

"Wow! So basically, the noise is to get our attention, so we can call the nurse?" Angel interrupted.

"Yes." Jane agreed. "You're a very smart girl!" Jane told Angel

"I know. Thank you, Mommy." Angel shrugged.

Jane and Jide made eye contact and smiled.

The first six days of chemotherapy went without any noted adverse event. The last day of chemotherapy, was a Sunday. Saturdays were Jane's day away from the hospital. She always spent the day with Angel at home. Jide was in charge on Saturdays. He spent the whole day with Gabe.

Although Angel stayed connected with Jane and Gabe via facetime and frequent hospital visits, her parents needed to make sure that she did not miss out on spending quality time with her mother.

Girl's time, involved redoing Angel's hair, making her favorite meals, watching her favorite television show and going to her favorite park. Angel needed normalcy in her life.

Returning to the hospital room that Sunday, Jane was relieved to see her boys laying on the bed and watching television. "How is Gabe doing?" She asked, looking him over from head to toe.

"He just received his last dose of chemotherapy and it seems uneventful." Jide replied.

Jane smiled. "How are you doing Gabe?"

"Good." he responded in his usual one-word answers.

"Is that hives on his face? Jane asked alarmed.

White patches where beginning to appear all over Gabe's body.

Jide pressed the nurse's call bell immediately.

Chapter Twenty-nine

The Allergic Reaction

The nurse arrived and paged the nurse practitioner on duty. Gabe was having an allergic reaction to the last and highest dose of his chemotherapy. The reaction was common with the drug and was expected. The appropriate medication was administered and the hives slowly disappeared. Over the next twelve hours; the hives played hide and seek. They would show up, he would get re-medicated and then, they slowly disappear.

With Gabe's initial allergic reaction, he received diphenhydramine. Jane and Jide soon realized that it made Gabe extremely agitated. He was frustrated with the predicament that he found himself in. He scratched, clawed and screamed. Jane wept silently. Together with Jide, they made a mental note to ask for an alternative medication.

The next day was a chemotherapy free day. Everyone was relieved to have a bit of rest.

Chapter Thirty

Transplant Day

Transplant day was a day like none other. A few morning nurses set up all medications required; in case of any emergency, during the procedure. A seasoned nurse practitioner came in to make sure that everything was setup as required. The transplant team came into the room, to make sure that nothing was amiss and every monitoring device was functional. Angel's bone marrow was delivered to the room in an infusion bag. Gabe received the bone marrow transplant via an intravenous infusion.

Jane watched closely as the fluid slowly drained into Gabe. She observed him closely to see if there were any sudden physical changes. There was no physical change, but Jane knew a momentous event when she saw one. On this day, Gabe was reborn.

Now, it was time for Gabe's body to start making new cells using Angel's bone marrow.

Chapter Thirty-one

After Chemotherapy

The weeks following the transplant were spent watching and waiting. Gabe was monitored very closely and many precautions were taken to prevent chemotherapy induced side effects.

The adverse effects from chemotherapy are usually seen in rapidly shedding cells in the body. Jane was expecting these side effects to show up a little over a week after chemotherapy. Gabe brushed every day with a disposal sponge. He rinsed his mouth and swallowed an antifungal agent to prevent painful sores in the mouth; oral thrush. Thankfully, he never got an oral infection. The food and nutrition department sent a menu every day. Gabe had fun deciding what he wanted to eat and drink the following day. His appetite remained unchanged throughout the treatment.

Initially, Jane did not want to put any diaper on Gabe. But after the first incident of bedwetting, she conceded.

"Why do I have to wear diapers?" Gabe protested.

"It's so you don't have to worry so much about waking up at night to pee." Jane responded.

"Don't worry Gabe. As soon as we get home, you can go back to your underwear." Jane reassured him.

"Ok." He said. Accepting the explanation.

The decision to use diapers also made it easier for the nurse to document his urine output.

Two weeks after chemotherapy, Gabe's skin became very itchy. With no rash in sight, everyone began to trouble shoot the cause for this sudden discomfort.

"I have been using hydrophilic ointment for his skin since he was born." Jane responded to the nurse's suggestion that Gabe might be allergic to his body cream.

The next day, they discovered that his hair was falling out from the back of his head. The buzz cut he received prior to admission made it hard to notice at first. However, short hair spikes were all over his pillowcase and the back of his shirt.

"Why is my hair falling?" Gabe asked Jane that afternoon.

"It's falling out, to make room for a fresh batch of hair." She answered, trying very hard to sound unaffected.

"Ok, Mummy." he said focusing on his Ninja Legend game.

The next day Jide came to visit. He was very distraught to see that Gabe was losing his hair.

Noticing the change in Jide, Jane walked to the bathroom and signaled for him to follow.

"Jide, do not give him that look!" She said.

"What look?" He asked confused.

"The look of pity." She responded.

"Don't you know that children pick up energy easily?" She asked.

"You can cry in this bathroom; like I do, but once you enter his room, you have to be cheerful." She smiled, as if to show him, how easy it was to be cheerful.

"You are right" Jide said.

He noticed that Jane was very stressed, but masked it with a calm facade. She declined going to the once weekly parent's meeting with the psychologist, because she was afraid to leave Gabe's side. Jide decided to bring Jane her favorite meal the next day. He knew that Jane did not want to dine out while at the hospital. She always ate Gabe's leftovers.

Returning to Gabe's room, Jide smiled at his son.

Together they discussed Gabe's itching and resolved that he needed another haircut.

They consulted with the transplant team, to see if Gabe could get another haircut. His clotting factors where still within normal limits; there was no risk of bleeding, so the hair cut was approved. After the haircut, Gabe walked into the shower with Jane pushing his medication stand behind him. The area surrounding his central line was covered with plastic and taped down, to prevent it from getting wet. Once he received a warm shower, the mysterious itching disappeared.

Evening shower, became a part of Gabe's bedtime routine. Every night at seven, Jane would dim the lights. Turn on the flashing star lights, spray a fresh smelling mist in the air and give Gabe a warm shower. She puts on his favorite show and set the television to sleep in two hours. Tucked in his bed, Gabe always fell asleep comfortably.

Soon, his skin started to darken, Jane continued to apply the hydrophilic ointment to his skin. One day, Jane noticed a slur in Gabe's speech. She watched him closely and realized that he seemed to have an excess amount of saliva in his mouth. The nurses had placed a suction device by his bedside at the beginning of the treatment. Jane called the nurse to show her how to properly use the device.

"It is as easy as flipping a switch." The nurse said.

"All he has to do is put it in his mouth and keep his mouth closed. It sucks out all the excess saliva."

Gabe started using the oral suction right away and soon it became a fun toy. In less than a week, the increased sputum phase passed.

Actually, Jane was not too sure when it ended. She noted that Gabe was trying to use the suction to clean his bed!

Despite these side effects, every morning Gabe got out of his bed and asked Jane to roll the heavy medication stand behind him, as he walked to the bay window in his room. Thanks to child life department, he had a huge cardboard house to play inside, with his toys.

When he got tired of playing by himself or with Jane, he played with the numerous hospital volunteers that stopped by. He especially loved when Angel dropped by to visit him.

Chapter Thirty-two

No More Immune System

Every morning, Jane would wake up before the nurses changed shifts, to shower and put on fresh clothing.

Gazing out of the window, she scribbled her thoughts in her journal as she ate some of Gabe's left-over food or cold cereal.

She made sure Gabe's room smelt fresh, all his toys were wiped down with bleach and placed out of the way; so that the housekeeping lady could work efficiently. Keeping the room clean, is key to preventing infections.

Soon, Gabe was completely immune compromised, his white blood count, platelets, you name it, was zero. Angel could no longer visit. This was to prevent her from inevitably bringing in any infections from the playground. They were content with facetiming each other daily.

Gabe received a plasma infusion, as his bone marrow worked hard to accept Angel's donation. Waiting; like Mrs. Gray said, was the hardest part. Blood was drawn early every morning to monitor his complete blood counts and electrolytes.

Gabe energy level remained unaltered. A few of his favorite visitors from the hospital's child life department were the art lady and the music man. He had given up his drum lessons to start his treatment, so he was very happy to strum the guitar strings.

Chapter Thirty-three

Central Line Mishap

From the onset of his treatment, Gabe's energy level never decreased. He would jump, run and roll with all the lines attached to him. The lines were heavy so they twisted as he rolled around. On one of these occasions, one of the branches developed a small tear and he began to bleed out.

"Mummy;" he spoke calmly, "I am wet."

Jane ran over and inspected the lines. She was shocked to see blood seeping out. Her heart sank to the pit of her stomach.

Dashing across the room, she pressed the nurse's call button. Remembering that Gabe's nurse was on a short break, she ran to the nurse's station to call the covering nurse.

The nurse came in swiftly and clamped the line. Then she dialed for the lines repair team. If the line could not be repaired, Gabe would have to go into the operating room to have the current line removed and replaced.

It had been such a good day. Gabe had been playing quietly by himself on the sofa bed.

"Why now?" Jane agonized. She was truly scared.

Gabe had to move from the sofa to his bed. He had to lay flat and hold still, so his nurse could assess the damage. Gabe did not want to lay still for the area to be assessed, he was alarmed. Jane was very worried and for once, Gabe looked at his mother's face and saw panic in her eyes.

He was twisting, turning and screaming. Silent tears fell down Jane's cheeks as she held him down, so that the nurse could remove the sterile tape that was covering the insertion point. His skin was sensitive underneath the sterile tape. The wipe used to clean the area was very cold and it stung him a bit.

After the assessment, it was determined that the line could be repaired. Once the line was repaired, Gabe calmed down.

Later that day, Jane spoke to Gabe to find out how he was feeling.

"Why did you cry so much?" She asked.

"The wipe was too cold, it burnt me and I don't like being held down." He replied,

"I'm so very sorry" cooed Jane; wrapping Gabe in a big hug and kissing his forehead.

"We could not waste any time," she continued.

"Don't do that again, Mummy." He admonished.

"I won't." She promised, praying that she would not have to live through the experience again.

Laying exhausted on the bed that night, Jane had to retell the entire story to Jide and Loveline. They all thanked God that the day ended on a good note.

Reflecting on the day's incident, Jane realized that she got an impromptu lesson on how to handle any tear to his central line. This gave her some peace of mind.

"Thank God this happened while we were still here in the hospital." She told Jide later.

"Should this happen at home, I will not panic again."

Chapter Thirty-four

Ready to go Home

As Gabe's bone marrow continued to regain its normal function, the plan was to convert most of his medications from the intravenous route to the oral route. This would make it easier for him to take his medication once he was discharged. He had to be discharged on two intravenous medications.

These medications did not taste very pleasant. With the chemotherapy and bone marrow transplant, Gabe had experienced some changes to his taste buds. He abhorred certain smells and did not like the look of any of his oral medications. The child life team tried to teach him how to swallow tablets, but he did not show much interest. Jane decided that she would handle this part of the process.

"With treats and constant pleading, I'm sure I can get him to take all his medications on time." She reassured the transplant team.

Jane had never shed so much tears in her life. She begged, cajoled, and bribed Gabe, just to get him to take his medications.

"Of what use is a transplant, if one does not take the medications to prevent rejection?" She would mutter to herself in frustration. She resolved that no matter what happens, Gabe will take his medication as scheduled. She was a mother on a mission!

Jide tried to help her once. He quickly realized that he did not have the patience needed, to undertake such a task. Angel also encouraged her little brother to take his medication. Medication time was a family affair. Gabe had been through so much, the least they could do, was to be very patient with him. Eventually, he took them promptly enough to be discharged.

Gabe was discharged with lots of precautions; to ensure that he did not get any infection, as his body continued to make the steady journey to regain its full function. Everything he ate had to be prepared at very high temperatures. Fruits had to be properly handled and peeled. He also had other restrictions. This ranged from zero exposure to sick people and crowds, to wearing masks virtually everywhere. There were numerous appointments each week for physical examination and blood work. Once a week, a visiting nurse came by the house, to make sure that his lines where functional and flushed.

In their hearts, Jane and Jide believed that Gabe was cured.

Jane became a cleaning lady at home. She white washed the walls with bleach wipes, mopped the floors multiple times daily and placed hand sanitizers at every corner of the house. No guests were allowed to visit Gabe except for his immediate family. She administered his intravenous medications every night and flushed all his lines; like she was taught to do by his hospital nurse.

Clearly, she could not keep this up once she returned to work, but she did not have to. She was scheduled to go back to work just when Gabe's isolation period ended.

Gabe was very excited to be home again. Angel came back home from her grandparent's home and reigned as Gabe's biggest cheerleader, encouraging him to down his "yucky" medications; as he loved to call them. Angel assumed a second "mother" role, bossing him around and reporting any changes to her parents.

Chapter Thirty-five

Out-Patient Clinic

Initially after discharge, they went to the outpatient clinic, multiple times a week. Over time, the days in-between visits slowly increased to once a year. Each visit requires a blood draw and a thorough physical exam. Gabe was no longer indifferent to needles, but he was brave. Once the central line was removed; less than six weeks after discharge, Jane and Jide were relieved.

Each day that passed, brought healing to Gabe's body. Within a couple of months, his hair was full of fluffy hair. As the weather cooled, Gabe caught a respiratory virus. Thankfully, his body was strong enough to fight and overcome it. His blood work soon normalized and his medications were discontinued as scheduled.

At Gabe's one-year post-transplant hospital visit, an extensive medical workup was done; just like the pre-transplant tests. All results came back within normal limits. He had gone from having sickle cell disease to having the sickle cell trait. He was cured!

Chapter Thirty-six

Life after Transplant

Jane worried that Gabe would be a handful at school. However, he gained maturity there. He worked very hard, landing on the math honor roll his first term and the principal's honor roll by the end of kindergarten. Some days, he says he wants to be a surgeon and on other days a ninja. Jane and Jide always look at each other and smile.

Two years post-transplant, he continues to thrive. Getting revaccinated, proves to be his biggest challenge, since all his immunity was wiped out with chemotherapy. This means that he gets three or four injections during his vaccination appointment. In typical Gabe fashion, he takes it all in stride.

Gabe has already forgotten the details surrounding the transplant. He may have forgotten about all the time he spent in isolation in the hospital, but he has not forgotten what his sister did for him. He has a deep sense of gratitude and unparalleled dedication for Angel.

Gabe's story is written to make sure he never forgets. It is written to spread a message of hope and most importantly, it is written to create awareness. Often times, family members, healthcare workers and the general public, do not know much about sickle cell disease. The pain, depression, and anxiety associated with the disease is misunderstood. Raising awareness removes the stigma associated with sickle cell disease. Once the etiology and pathophysiology of the disease is truly understood, it easier to provide care and support.

Finally, many individuals do not know that they carry the sickle cell trait. This should never be the case.

Do you know your genotype?

The good news is that we have a cure! Researchers continue to strive to create different and hopefully easier ways to attain it.

If you are affected by this disease, do not give up. Arm yourself with knowledgeable healthcare professionals. Let your voice be heard. Develop a healthy eating habit, know your physical, emotional and psychological limits. Be sure to get all recommended vaccines. Most importantly love completely, smile often and live your best life.

About the Author

Dr. Nancy Chinyere Butler has practiced in the retail pharmacy setting; in New York City, for over a decade and she loves it. She is a strong believer in sharing experiences to help make the world a healthier place.

When she is not at work, she loves spending time with her family, swimming, traveling, dinning with friends, meeting new people, listening to podcasts, music, reading romantic novels and writing.

Did you learn anything new about sickle cell disease from this novel? Be sure to share with others.

Share your thoughts with the author on Instagram #chy_butler.

Do not forget to leave a review on amazon.